Table of Contents

Absence Seizures

An absence seizure is a type of seizure that is characterized by a sudden and brief moment of unconsciousness. These seizures are most common in children. Usually it will appear that the individual is daydreaming and simply staring off into space. The type of seizure is much milder than other types of seizures, but they can still be dangerous. Children that experience absence seizures should be closely supervised when bathing or swimming as a lapse in consciousness could result in drowning.

Absence seizures can easily be treated though. Determining which medication is correct for the individual can be a little perplexing at times. Zarontin, Depakene, and Lamactil are the most commonly prescribed medications for absence seizures. It is very important for the patients to continue taking anti-seizure medications for up to two years after the last incident because relapsing is very common in many patients.

Allergic to the Cold

It seems very strange to seriously say that one is allergic to the cold. However, this may not be far from the truth. It seems that, in some individuals, the body has a unique reaction to skin exposure to low temperatures. In certain cases, the body reacts differently to the cold by releasing histamine and various other chemicals into the skin. These histamines are the same ones associated in common allergies. The histamines typically cause urticaria which is also known as cold hives.

The causes for these reactions in certain people is not currently clear, but there is a regular occurrence in most cases. Often, people with these allergies have overly-sensitive histamine containing skin cells. It seems that there may be a connection between the skin cells and the cold hives.

It is very important for individuals with these kinds of reactions to cold to avoid exposure to cold temperatures. Submersion in cold water could
have severe consequences for the individuals suffering from these types of allergies. The reactions could be fatal in some instances of great overexposure to the cold.

Acute Respiratory Distress

Acute respiratory distress syndrome is a failure of the respiratory system which can occur rather quickly. It occurs when the the air sacs of the lungs, known as the aveoli, suddenly fill up with fluids. This deprives your body of oxygen and breathing becomes very difficult in a short length of time. The condition usually occurs in individuals who are extremely ill or have severe injuries. Between twenty-five to forty percent of people who experience ARDS do not survive. Those who do survive typically do not regain full use of their lungs for up to a full year.

ARDS is usually indicated by

a shortness of breath, difficulty breathing, extreme fatigue, and a weak pulse. ARDS is usually accompanied by another life-threatening condition so it requires immediate medical attention. The treatment for ARDS consists of providing the body with much needed oxygen. This is typically accomplished through means of a ventilator or supplemental oxygen. Patients are given a varied of medications to include pain relievers, anticoagulants, corticosteroids, and even sedatives. There is hope in most case for the individual to recover from the condition. The prognosis is highly dependent on what other factors attributed to the condition.

A different type of infertility

As ridiculous as it may seem, there actually are rare medical cases in which individual have been allergic to semen. In actuality, they are allergic to certain proteins in the semen. The allergy to the semen proteins is not the direct cause for infertility in such cases, but the prevenative measures also prevent pregnacies. The most common way to prevent allergic reactions in semen allergies is the use of a condom which is also prevents pregnacy. In most cases, burning and itching along with swelling of the outer vaginal area are the common reactions to the allergies. In some cases, individual have broken out into hives and also had difficulty breathing.

If the symptoms occur that would lead one to think they might have allergic reactions, it is best to have an allergy test to determine if semen allergies are the correct diagnosis. Pregnancy would still be possible in the cases of semen allergies. In severe cases, one can consult their doctor to see if artificial insemination or in vitro fertilization would be necessary for the individual to have children.

Acanthosis Nigricans

Acanthosis nigricans is a skin condition characterized by dark, thick, velvety skin in parts of the body such as the armpits, groin, and neck. The condition usually causes individuals to be very concerned with the appearance of their skin. The condition is a gradual darkening of the skin and, in a few rare cases, can be itchy.

The condition is usually associated with patients who have type 2 diabetes or are excessively overweight. High levels of insulin have been known to cause changes to the body's skin conditions. In some cases, the arcanthosis nigricans has been associated with heredity. Several cases have been linked to certain medications like oral contraceptives, human growth hormone, and large doses of niacin. Very rarely is the condition related to cancer.

There is no specific treatment for the condition, but there are a few ways to help those who have concerns about their skin's condition. Doctors can prescribe lotions like tretinoin to lighten the affected areas. There are also some oral medications like isotretinoin which help improve the condition. It has also been advised to take fish oil supplements for the condition. In addition, for those who wish, laser therapy can reduce the affected areas in most cases.

Vulvodynia

Vulvodynia is a medical condition that is commonly unreported by many women who experience it. The condition is noted by symptoms that result in vaginal pain around the areas around the vaginal opening. Many women note burning and itching sensations along with rawness and throbbing that can last for months or years. The irritations and pain can be continuous or intermittent. In most cases, the feelings will come on very suddenly and vanish just as suddenly. The tissue around the area may appear to be inflamed or even swollen. This will cause intercourse to be very unpleasant.

Vulvodynia has been attributed to a variety of causes. These causes include injury and nerve damage to the area around the vulva, chronic vaginal infections, allergies, muscle spasms, and estrogen level fluctuations as a result of female menopause. The condition is not normally a sign of cancer in most situations.

Women do not normally report the signs of the condition, but they should. As many as one in six women experience vulvodynia. The condition is actually common and nothing to be ashamed of. There are a variety of medications available to treat the symptoms associated with the condition. The medications include amitriptyline, desipramine (Norpramin), and nortriptyline (Aventyl, Pamelor). Also, there are options for physical therapy treatments and topical creams to relieve the pain associated with vulvodynia.

Vaginal Atrophy

The inflammation and thinning of the vaginal walls due to a drop in the levels of estrogen is called vaginal atrophy. The condition is seen during female menopause in most cases, but the condition has also occurred in cases of women who have developed breast cancer. The condition is caused by decreases in estrogen levels so it could occur at any time in which the estrogen levels have dropped for some reason.

The condition has very noticeable symptoms which include vaginal dryness and burning, watery discharges from the vaginal area, urinary tract infections with burning urination, and pain during intercourse. In many cases, a tightening and shortening of the vaginal canal has also been noted. The condition is typically experience by about half of women during menopause. Therefore, it is not out of the ordinary to experience the condition. If you experience the symptoms, let your doctor know so that the condition can be treated.

Since the condition makes sexual intercourse very painful, women tend to loose interest and drastically decrease their sex drive. On the bright side, the condition is easily treated. The treatment for vaginal atrophy usually consists of estrogen creams, tablets, or sometimes an estrogen ring that can be inserted in the upper area of the vagina. In most cases, improvements in the condition have been noted in a few weeks. Some cases take a little longer, but the condition is easily treated.

Crohn's Disease

Crohn's disease is a condition which has severe effects on the gastrointestinal tract. The condition usually begins in the lower part of the small intestine or the colon and can spread throughout the entire tract. The disease starts as an inflammation of the gastrointestinal tract and can lead to symptoms that can be life-threatening. There is no clear evidence that has pointed to a specific cause of Crohn's disease, but many researchers believe that it is either caused by the immune systems reaction to specific microbes or by heredity. Regardless of the causes of Crohn's disease, the condition can be very dangerous if left untreated.

Crohn's disease is noted by severe

abdominal pains, blood in the stool, chronic diarrhea, and unexplainable fevers. When these symptoms are noticed, it would be best to see your doctor. Typically, your family doctor will refer you to a gastrointestinal specialist when such symptoms are noticed. The specialist will be able to verify if Crohn's disease is the cause of the symptoms. Some of the dangers of untreated Crohn's disease include gastrointestinal tract obstructions, ulcers, fistulas (which can be life-threatening if untreated), anal fissures, and malnutrition.

Crohn's disease is treated with a mixture of medications or surgery. A patient will receive three types of medications for Crohn's disease which include anti-inflammatory drugs, immune system suppressors, and antibiotics. In addition, patients might also be given anti-diarrheal drugs, laxatives, pain relievers, iron supplements, or various other vitamin supplements depending on their individual cases. If diet, exercise, and medications do not improve the patient's condition, surgery is an option for patients. The most common surgery that Crohn's disease patients undergo is strictureplasty. During the operation, a section of the individual's intestines are widen to allow food to pass through more easily. Usually, the benefits are only temporary. It is very common for patients that undergo surgery to need the operation repeated. For best results, patients need to continue their prescribed medications after surgery.

Q Fever

Q fever is a virus that I was unfortunate enough to learn about while deployed to Iraq with US military. The condition is very similar to aseptic meningitis by its noticeable symptoms. The patient usually will experience a persistent fever accompanied with sever headaches and a rash that first appears on his extremities and then will spread to the torso. The fever will break on a daily basis but then come back the following day. The headache will be consistent throughout the duration of the condition. In addition, the patient will typically experience a loss of appetite along with nausea and vomiting. The condition can be acute or chronic in its nature as it is common for the patient to relapse repeatedly. Typically, diagnosis can be confirmed by means of obtaining spinal fluid. The treatment for the condition consists of Doxcysilin given to the patient twice a day for three weeks. Pain medication such as Tylenol can be given for the headache and associated fatigue that patient experiences due to the condition.

Q fever is still being studied by western doctors. Research is in its early stages concerning the condition. Over recent years, many individuals that have been deployed to the Middle East have experienced the disease. Q fever can be a very serious condition if not treated. When its symptoms are experienced it is best to seek medical treat as soon as possible.

Sickle Cell Anemia

Sickle cell anemia is a condition that is caused by a genetice l mutation. The condition affects African-Americans and those of northern Mediterranean ancestry. The prevalence of the condition is in 1 out of 600 individuals and occurs when both parents have the gene needed. Sickle cell anemia is caused by the altered shape of red blood cell which results in the cells having a crescent shape.

The symptoms of sickle cell anemia include chronic fatigue, difficulty breathing during exercise, joint swelling, and paleness. A diagnosis can be concluded through lab tests and by looking at one's family history. Lab tests will show decreased hemoglobin and hematocrit along with lower red blood cell counts. There will be an increase in the white blood cell and platelet count also. Sickle cell anemia is typically treated with antibiotics, vaccinations, and analgesics during a crisis time. It is important for patients with sickle cell anemia to maintain a diet with foods high in folic acid, maintain hydration, rest, and exercise regularly.

Dementia.

Dementia is a concern for many people as a large portion of the population is approaching old age. A person who has dementia must show impairments in memory. Usually this begins with having trouble remembering new information and then progresses to loss of older memories. Additionally, individuals suffering from dementia will have at least one other cognitive deficit such as aphasia, apraxia, agnosia, or a disturbance of executive functioning.

Aphasia is a difficulty in communicating. There are two common types of aphasias. Broca's Aphasia is referred to as an expressive aphasia because the person will understand you, but they will have difficulty communicating to you. This is not due to a speech impediment. They simply have trouble communicating what they want to say. The second type of aphasia is Wernicke's Aphasia. This is considered a receptive type of aphasia. In this case, the individual is unable to understand what is being conveyed to them even though their hearing is fine. Typically, what they hear sounds like a "word salad" that does not make sense. They will still be able to communicate to you though.

The second cognitive deficit is apraxia. Apraxia is an impairment of motor functions or movements. This can be seen as an impairment of gross motor movement which can be seen large movements such as walking and running. Additionally, fine motor movements can be impaired which include things such as writing and precise small movements. Often fine motor apraxia that affects the vocal cords can be confused with aphasia, but it is more correctly identified as apraxia.

The third type of cognitive deficit is agnosia. Agnosia is an inability to identify things such as people, objects, and other items that a person would normally have an easy time identifying. Propoagnosia is the inability to remember faces and names of people. A humorous example is that of the man who mistook his wife for a hat and actually attempted put his wife on his head.

The impairments of executive functioning can be seen as impairments in the person's ability to plan things. These individuals may have difficulty put clothing on in the correct order or planning the day's activities in a logical manner. For instance, the person may have confuse the correct steps needed to return home and take a scenic route unnecessarily causing a fifteen minute trip to take two hours.

Munchhausen syndrome

Munchhausen syndrome-
Munchhausen syndrome is a condition in
which a person will fake illness in order to
get the attention of others. The person will
typically go to great lengths to ensure that
they will appear ill. The individual will
create numerous medical expenses. They
will undergo surgeries and procedures. The
will take medicine that will otherwise be
dangerous to them. The difficult thing about
diagnosing Munchhausen syndrome is that a
patient will abruptly change doctors and
hospitals if they feel their true disorder is
about to be revealed.

Munchhausen syndrome by proxy-
Munchhausen by proxy can actually be

potentially more dangerous
than regular Munchhausen. The classic
example of this condition was a mother
whose daughter became ill suddenly and
without reason. The daughter was convinced
by the mother's reactions and believes that
there was something wrong with her. The
daughter underwent numerous tests and
operations as a result of the mother's belief
that there was something wrong with the
child. When the mother was not present the
daughter did not present any of the
symptoms or problems. This kind of
situation can easily be construed as child
abuse. In most of the cases, it is actually
determined that the parents coaching of the
child to feign such illnesses and conditions
and undergo operations to correct a non-

existent condition is, in fact, child abuse. The driving factor for the parent is typically to get the attention or pity of other individuals due to the circumstance of having an ill child and the parent having to take on such a burden of taking care of such a child.

Gender Identity Disorder

In the following, I have outlined the criteria for Gender Identity Disorder. Firstly, a strong and persistent cross-gender identification must be present.
In children, they will repeatedly state a desire to be or insist that they are the other sex. In boys, a preference for cross-dressing in female attire will manifest. In girls, they will insist on wearing stereotypical masculine clothing. A strong and persistent preference for cross-sex roles in make believe play or persistent fantasies of being the other sex will occur in children. They will show intense desire to participate in the stereotypical games and pastimes of the

other sex. The child will also show a strong preference for playmates of the other sex.

In adolescents and adults, the disturbance is manifested by symptoms such as stated desire to be the other sex, frequent passing as the other sex, and/or a desire to live and be treated as the other sex. The individual will show a persistent discomfort with his or her sex and display a sense of inappropriateness in the gender role of that sex. In boys, this could be in the form of assertion that his penis or testes are disgusting or that it would be better not to have a penis. Also the boy may reject stereotypical male toys, games, and activities. Girls will reject the concept of urinating in a sitting position. She will assert that she will grow a penis. Also she may state that she does not want to grow breasts or menstruate. In adolescents and adults, a preoccupation with getting rid of primary and secondary

gender characteristics through procedures to physically alter sexual characteristics to stimulate others in a way that one of the other gender would may be present.

www.ingramcontent.com/pod-product-compliance
Lightning Source LLC
Chambersburg PA
CBHW021448170526
45164CB00001B/438